FIT MIND
BRYAN & STEPHANIE VIGNERY

Keep FIT MIND near your workstation.

Let a positive way of looking at life set your mind for the challenges and victories you will see today.

Copyright © 2020 by Bryan & Stephanie Vignery

Fit Mind
By Bryan & Stephanie Vignery

ISBN-13: 987-1-7345640-0-6

All rights reserved. This book may not be reproduced in whole or in part in any form or format without permission in writing from the author, except for brief quotations in a review.

Where possible, quotations are attributed to their source. All rights reserved by the author or rights holder.

Bible quotation marked (CSB) is taken from The Christian Standard Bible. Copyright © 2017 by Holman Bible Publishers. Used by permission. Christian Standard Bible®, and CSB® are federally registered trademarks of Holman Bible Publishers, all rights reserved.

FIT MIND

DAY ONE

"I am not what happened to me.
I am what I choose to become."

– *Carl Jung*

Life is all about choices. Will we let our past continue into our future, or will we choose to acknowledge our past and receive healing from it?

Depending on the answer, we might actually begin to build the life we were created to enjoy.

FIT MIND

FIT MIND

DAY TWO

You don't get what you wish for,
you get what you work for.

Are you waiting, hoping, and wishing for things in your life to change?

Changes only happen when we take action to make them happen. The most powerful person standing in the way of what you want from life

... is you!

DAY 2

FIT MIND

FIT MIND

DAY THREE

"Look in the mirror.
That's your competition."

What do you see when you look at yourself?

Some see beauty and value; others see sadness, anger, or lack of worth. Whatever you see, know this: we will be our own worst critic until we start to see ourselves through the eyes of our Maker.

FIT MIND

FIT MIND

DAY FOUR

"Change doesn't always require growth,
but growth always requires change."

Without change, growth is impossible. A decision to grow is a decision to change—a worthwhile and powerful decision to make.

Will you step out of your comfort zone and start today to change and grow?

FIT MIND

DAY FIVE

> "You don't have to be great to start,
> but you have to start to be great."
>
> *– Zig Ziglar*

Starting, of course, is the hardest part. Once we start, however, we are halfway there to being glad we did. We weren't created to be ordinary; we were created to be extraordinary.

Just begin and embrace the journey God has for you.

FIT MIND

FIT MIND

DAY SIX

"The body achieves
what the mind believes."

*– Inspired by Napoleon Hill's
"Whatever the mind can conceive
and believe, the mind can achieve."*

Do you believe you can reach your health goals?

Henry Ford once said, "Whether you think you can or think you can't, you're right." So believe in your ability. Once your mindset changes, everything on the outside will change along with it.

FIT MIND

FIT MIND

DAY SEVEN

"Your mind is a powerful thing.
When you fill it with positive thoughts,
your life will start to change."

Finding the negative in life is easy. When we have a negative focus, negative seems to happen. But, when we focus on things we can be grateful for, we will notice the positive things.

And it is those things which reveal the person God created us to be.

DAY 7

FIT MIND

DAY EIGHT

FIT MIND

"Whatever you're thinking, think bigger."

– *Tony Hsieh*

Do not limit what God can do. Think big! Anything is possible with God.

FIT MIND

DAY 8

FIT MIND

DAY NINE

"When I lost all of my excuses,
I found all my results."

When an achievement is important to us, we will find a way. If not, we will find excuses. Don't allow opportunities to pass you by because of excuses. Create a list of your priorities.

Remember, God can make a way where there seems to be no way.

FIT MIND

DAY TEN

"Don't wait until you reach your goal
to be proud of yourself.
Be proud of every step you take."

The journey is all about progress, not perfection. We cannot expect changes overnight. However, when we decide that we want to accomplish a goal, and we give it 100% effort, over time, we can be happy with the journey.

FIT MIND

DAY ELEVEN

FIT MIND

"Being happy doesn't mean that
everything is perfect.
It means you've decided
to look beyond the imperfections."

– Gerard Way

No one but God is perfect. When we begin to realize that it is not about achieving perfection, life will be more enjoyable.

Successful people do not become successful by being perfect but by learning from imperfections.

FIT MIND

DAY 11

DAY TWELVE

"Don't let someone who gave up
on their dreams
talk you out of going after yours."

– *Zig Ziglar*

When you hear those voices—all around you or inside you—telling you that you can't reach the goal or dream you desire, consider the source. Don't give your power away.

Those goals and dreams just may be God-given.

FIT MIND

DAY THIRTEEN

FIT MIND

"Never give up on a dream
just because of the time it will take
to accomplish it.
The time will pass anyway."

– Earl Nightingale

God doesn't give us a dream unless He knows we have the ability to accomplish it. And because He wants us to accomplish it, He will continue to bring it to our mind until we have completed it.

God wants to give us desires and dreams.

DAY FOURTEEN

> "Failure is simply the opportunity
> to begin again,
> this time more intelligently."
>
> *– Henry Ford*

Thank God for second chances! Our biggest failures can be our most significant growth moments. Don't let failure hold you back. Fail forward!

FIT MIND

FIT MIND

DAY FIFTEEN

"Starting is more than half the battle.
You may fail, or you may succeed,
but either way,
jump in and enjoy the journey."

We should never give up on ourselves. God doesn't give up on us. Why should we?

Failure can become a springboard toward success when we allow ourselves to learn from the lessons it teaches.

FIT MIND

FIT MIND

DAY SIXTEEN

"Turn a setback into a comeback."

Forget the mistakes. Remember the lessons.

Every day is a new day.

FIT MIND

DAY 16

FIT MIND

DAY SEVENTEEN

"Your attitude, not your aptitude,
will determine your altitude."

– *Zig Ziglar*

What attitude am I wearing today?

When we are covered with "stinkin' thinkin'," not only do we bring others down, but we bring ourselves down. Instead, let's clothe ourselves with an "attitude of gratitude" and be thankful for what we have.

FIT MIND

DAY 17

FIT MIND

DAY EIGHTEEN

"Life has two rules:

#1 Never quit
#2 Always remember rule #1"

Never give up. Just think; when we quit, we could be missing an opportunity that is just around the corner. I firmly believe that if you start something, you must finish it.

Never give up ... ever!

FIT MIND

FIT MIND

DAY NINETEEN

"The moment you want to quit
is the moment
when you need to keep pushing."

Our mind will give up before our body does. Our body can do more than we think it can. When our mind tells our body to do something or to keep going, it will. Our mind is more powerful than we think it is.

FIT MIND

DAY TWENTY

"You never fail until you stop trying."

– *Albert Einstein*

There is no reason to run away from your challenges. Acknowledge them. Face them. Push through them. You will conquer them.

DAY 20

FIT MIND

FIT MIND

DAY TWENTY-ONE

"You can watch me,
mock me, block me, or join me.
What you cannot do is stop me."

With an unstoppable mindset and God on our side, we can do anything! What—or who—could possibly get in the way of creating the life we want and desire?

Is this the way you think?

FIT MIND

DAY TWENTY-TWO

FIT MIND

"To create 'Awesome' in your life,
you have to have a
'Make It Happen' mindset."

– Bryan Vignery

Our mind has a lot to do with what we create in our life. It really does come down to the choices we make.

FIT MIND

DAY 22

DAY TWENTY-THREE

FIT MIND

"Because He is, I AM!"

"I AM statements" are the things we say about ourselves ... to ourselves. They are key to how we live our lives.

No matter how we may feel, we must get rid of negative I AM statements and replace them with positive I AM statements.

FIT MIND

FIT MIND

DAY TWENTY-FOUR

"Always remember,
your focus determines your reality."

– *George Lucas*

What we feed will grow; what we starve will die. Look at what are you feeding in your life.

Is the fully-grown version worth it? If not, are you willing to step forward and make some sacrifices so you can get to where you truly desire to be?

FIT MIND

FIT MIND

DAY TWENTY-FIVE

"They say that life is a marathon. There are four-hundred, twenty-two 100-meter sprints in a marathon. Don't give up on one lost sprint."

– Bryan Vignery

Don't let the one small thing you didn't reach keep you from the one big thing you desire to reach!

FIT MIND

DAY 25

DAY TWENTY-SIX

FIT MIND

"No matter how you feel:
get up, dress up, show up,
and never give up."

– Genevieve Rhode

Giving less than 100% effort will give us less than 100% results. Arm yourself with a 'make it happen' mindset. Give it nothing less than 100%.

DAY 26

FIT MIND

DAY TWENTY-SEVEN

FIT MIND

"Smile often. Think positively. Give thanks. Laugh loudly. Love others. Dream big."

Life is too short. We should do each and every one of these simple things every day. When we do, it opens our heart to building a long and happy life.

FIT MIND

DAY TWENTY-EIGHT

"Today's actions are tomorrow's results."

Small daily habits create long-term lifestyle results. The habits that we act on daily predict the outcome of our mental, physical, emotional, and spiritual health.

FIT MIND

DAY TWENTY-NINE

FIT MIND

"When someone reacts,
they come from a place of fear;
when someone responds,
they come from a place of love."

– Bryan Vignery

If we want to create a peaceful environment around us, we have to choose to respond rather than react. When we respond, we lead from a position of love. Responding will change our environment.

People can't fight love.

DAY THIRTY

FIT MIND

"Have a blessed day ...
because the choice is yours!"

– *Bryan Vignery*

It is a beautiful thing that life is all about making our own choices. Some choices are good, of course, some, not so good. The key is to make choices that can bless someone else's life.

When we bless others, we will also be blessed.

FIT MIND

DAY THIRTY-ONE

"I didn't come this far
to only come this far."

[Jesus] asked his disciples, "Who do people say that the Son of Man is?" They replied, "Some say John the Baptist; others, Elijah; still others, Jeremiah or one of the prophets." "But you," he asked them, "who do you say that I am?"

(Matthew 16:13–15 CSB)

FIT MIND

www.ingramcontent.com/pod-product-compliance
Lightning Source LLC
Chambersburg PA
CBHW081126080526
44587CB00021B/3758